THE CANDIDA DIET COOKBOOK
FOR BEGINNERS

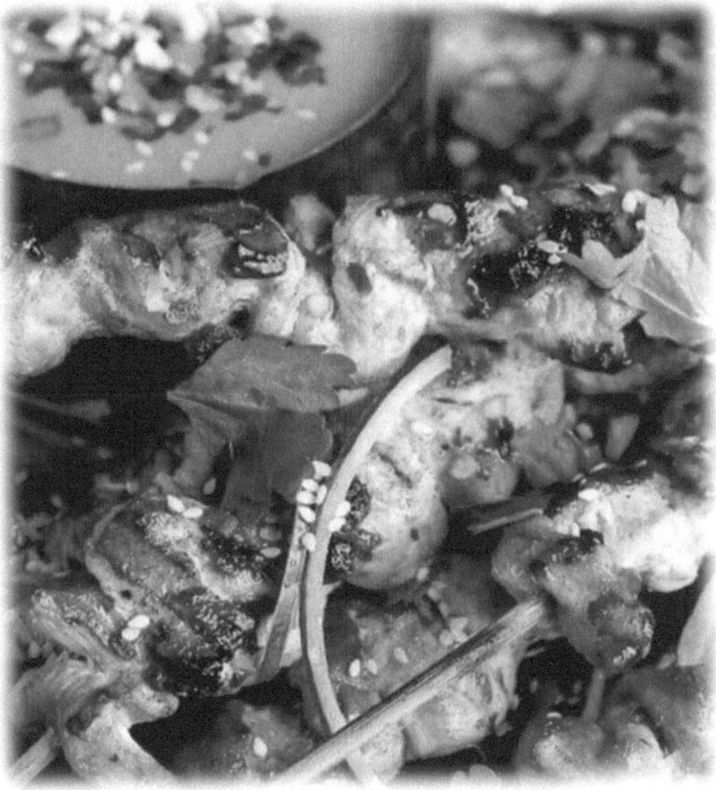

Nutritious Easy to Prepare Recipe To
Restore Your Gut Health

LAKEISHA   OWENS

TABLE OF CONTENT

INTRODUCTION

Candida, a yeast-like fungus that naturally resides in our body, can sometimes proliferate beyond healthy levels, leading to a myriad of uncomfortable symptoms and health issues. This book is crafted with the intent to provide you with the recipes needed to navigate this condition, aiming for a balanced gut flora and overall health improvement. Embarking on a diet to manage candida overgrowth can seem daunting at first, with various foods to avoid and new dietary principles to embrace. Within these pages, you'll find a curated selection of recipes that are not only tailored to be candida-friendly but are also designed to be delicious, satisfying, and easy to prepare. From hearty breakfasts and nutritious smoothies to satisfying main courses and safe, sweet treats, each recipe is crafted to ensure it meets the dietary requirements necessary to help manage candida overgrowth, emphasizing whole, unprocessed foods, healthy fats, and low glycemic ingredients.

Whether you're newly diagnosed with candida overgrowth, looking to prevent its occurrence, or simply aiming to adopt a healthier lifestyle, this cookbook provides the stepping stones towards achieving your health and wellness goals. As you turn the pages, remember that embarking on this dietary journey is a step towards taking control of your health. With each recipe and piece of advice, you're not just cooking; you're nurturing your body, fostering resilience, and opening the door to a more vibrant, energetic life.

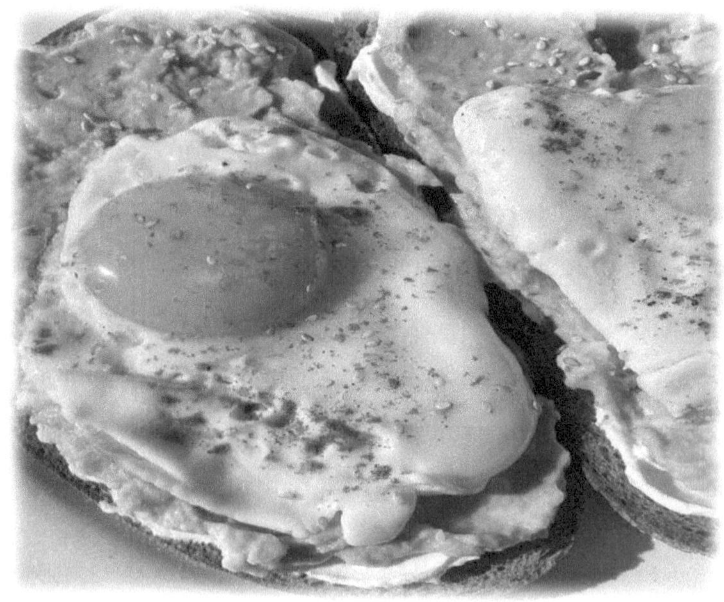

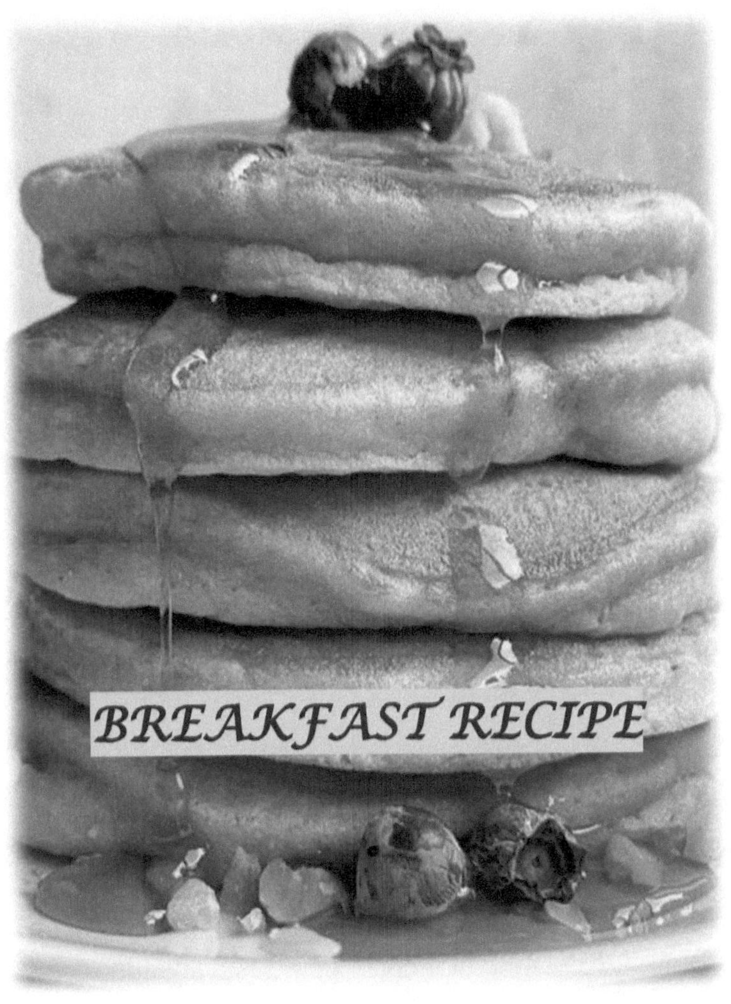
BREAKFAST RECIPE

RECIPE

Breakfast Recipe
Coconut Flour Pancakes

Ingredients:

4 tablespoons coconut flour
1 tablespoon of flaxseed combined with 3 tablespoons of water (flax egg).
1/2 cup unsweetened almond milk
1 teaspoon baking powder
1 teaspoon vanilla extract (ensure its sugar-free)
Coconut oil for cooking

Instructions:

Combine the ground flaxseed and water, and put aside for 5 minutes to thicken.

In a bowl, combine coconut flour and baking powder.

Stir in the flax egg, almond milk, and vanilla extract until the batter is smooth.

Heat a pan with a little coconut oil over medium heat.

Pour batter to form pancakes.

Cook until bubbles appear, then turn and finish until golden.

Serve warm.

Avocado & Egg Salad

Ingredients:

1 ripe avocado

2 hard-boiled eggs, chopped

1 tablespoon chopped chives

Lemon juice, to taste

Salt and pepper, to taste

Instructions:

Halve the avocado and remove the pit.

Scoop the flesh into a bowl.

Add the chopped eggs, chives, lemon juice, salt, and
pepper.

Mix gently until well combined.

Serve chilled.

Candida-Friendly Omelet

Ingredients:

2 eggs

1/2 cup spinach, chopped

2 tablespoons bell peppers, diced

1 tablespoon olive oil

Salt and pepper, to taste

Instructions:

Beat the eggs in a bowl.

Stir in the spinach and bell peppers.

Heat olive oil in a skillet over moderate heat.

Pour in the egg mixture, tilting the pan to spread evenly.

Cook until set, then fold the omelet in half.

Serve hot.

Almond Flour Porridge

Ingredients:

1/3 cup almond flour

1 cup unsweetened almond milk

1/2 teaspoon cinnamon

1 tablespoon almond butter

Stevia or monk fruit sweetener, to taste

Instructions:

In a pot, combine almond flour and almond milk.

Cook over moderate heat, stirring constantly to prevent lumps.

Once thickened, remove from heat and stir in cinnamon, almond butter, and sweetener.

Serve warm.

Green Detox Smoothie

Ingredients:

1 cup spinach

1/2 cucumber, chopped

1/4 avocado

1 tablespoon chia seeds

1 cup unsweetened coconut water

Lemon juice, to taste

Instructions:

Blend all ingredients until smooth.
Serve immediately.

Chia Seed Pudding

Ingredients:

3 tablespoons chia seeds
1 cup unsweetened almond milk
1/2 teaspoon vanilla extract (ensure its sugar-free)
Stevia or monk fruit sweetener, to taste
Cinnamon, for garnish

Instructions:

Mix chia seeds, almond milk, vanilla, and sweetener in a

bowl.

Refrigerate for at least 4 hours or overnight until it
thickens.
Serve with a sprinkle of cinnamon.

Herb-Infused Scrambled Eggs

Ingredients:

3 eggs

1 tablespoon fresh herbs (such as parsley, dill, or basil), chopped

1 tablespoon olive oil

Salt and pepper, to taste

Instructions:

Beat the eggs with salt, pepper, and fresh herbs.

Heat olive oil in a pan over moderate heat.

Add the egg mixture, cooking and stirring until the eggs are set.

Serve hot.

Zucchini Noodles with Avocado Sauce

Ingredients:

2 medium zucchinis, spiralized

1 ripe avocado

1/4 cup fresh basil leaves

2 tablespoons lemon juice

1 garlic clove

Salt and pepper, to taste

1 tablespoon olive oil

Instructions:

Blend avocado, basil, lemon juice, garlic, salt, and pepper until smooth.

Heat olive oil in a pan and briefly sauté the zucchini noodles for 1-2 minutes.

Remove from heat and mix with the avocado sauce.

Serve immediately.

Broccoli and Kale Breakfast Stir-Fry

Ingredients:

1 cup broccoli florets

1 cup kale, chopped

1 garlic clove, minced

2 tablespoons coconut oil

Salt and pepper, to taste

1 tablespoon pumpkin seeds

Instructions:

Heat coconut oil in a pan over moderate heat.

Add garlic and sauté until fragrant.

Add broccoli and kale, cooking until tender but still crisp.

Season with salt and pepper.

Garnish with pumpkin seeds before serving.

Cauliflower Rice Porridge

Ingredients:

2 cups cauliflower rice

1 cup unsweetened almond milk

1/2 teaspoon cinnamon

Stevia or monk fruit sweetener, to taste

1 tablespoon coconut oil

Instructions:

Heat coconut oil in a pan over moderate heat.

Add cauliflower rice, almond milk, and cinnamon.

Cook, stirring occasionally, until the mixture is creamy.

Sweeten to taste and serve warm.

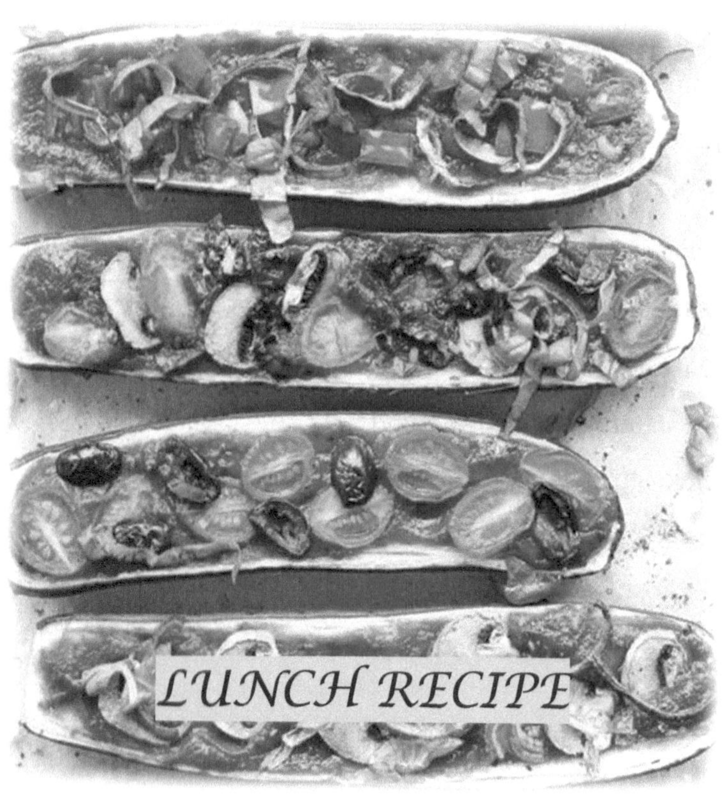

LUNCH RECIPE

LUNCH RECIPE

Grilled Chicken Salad with Lemon Dressing

Ingredients:

2 chicken breasts, grilled and sliced

4 cups mixed greens (spinach, arugula, lettuce)

1 cucumber, sliced

1/2 red bell pepper, sliced

1/4 cup olive oil

Juice of 1 lemon

Salt and pepper, to taste

Instructions:

In a large bowl, mix the greens, cucumber, and red bell pepper.

Whisk together olive oil, lemon juice, salt, and pepper to make the dressing.

Add the grilled chicken pieces to the salad.

Drizzle the dressing over the salad and gently mix before serving.

Cauliflower Rice Stir-Fry

Ingredients:

2 cups cauliflower rice

1 tablespoon coconut oil

1/2 cup broccoli florets

1/2 cup diced carrots

1/4 cup diced red bell pepper

2 tablespoons tamari or coconut aminos

1 teaspoon grated ginger

2 garlic cloves, minced

Instructions:

Heat coconut oil in a large skillet over moderate heat.

Add garlic and ginger, sautéing until fragrant.

Add the broccoli and carrots, cooking for about 5 minutes.

Stir in the cauliflower rice and red bell pepper, cooking for another 5-7 minutes.

Add tamari or coconut aminos, stir well, and serve hot.

Zucchini Boat Pizzas

Ingredients:

4 medium zucchinis, halved lengthwise

1 cup sugar-free tomato sauce

1 cup shredded mozzarella cheese (or a dairy-free

alternative)

1/2 cup sliced mushrooms

1/2 cup spinach, chopped

1 teaspoon oregano

Salt and pepper, to taste

Instructions:

Preheat your oven to 375°F (190°C).

Scoop out the center of each zucchini half to create a

"boat."

Spread tomato sauce inside each zucchini boat.

Top with cheese, mushrooms, and spinach.

Season with oregano, salt, and pepper.

Bake for 20–25 minutes, or until the zucchini is soft.

Serve hot.

Avocado Tuna Salad

Ingredients:

2 cans of tuna, drained

1 ripe avocado, mashed

1/4 cup diced celery

1/4 cup diced red onion

2 tablespoons lemon juice

Salt and pepper, to taste

Instructions:

In a bowl, combine the tuna and mashed avocado.

Add celery, red onion, and lemon juice.

Mix well.

Season with salt and pepper to taste.

Serve chilled with cucumber slices or lettuce wraps.

Turkey and Vegetable Skewers

Ingredients:

1 lb. (450g) turkey breast, cut into cubes

2 bell peppers, cut into pieces

1 zucchini, sliced

1 red onion, cut into chunks

2 tablespoons olive oil

1 teaspoon garlic powder

Salt and pepper, to taste

Instructions:

Preheat the grill to medium-high heat.

Thread turkey, bell peppers, zucchini, and red onion onto skewers.

Brush with olive oil and season with garlic powder, salt, and pepper.

Grill for 10-15 minutes, turning occasionally, until the turkey is cooked through.

Serve hot.

Creamy Coconut Spinach Soup

Ingredients:

4 cups spinach

1 can coconut milk

1 onion, diced

2 garlic cloves, minced

2 cups vegetable broth

1 tablespoon coconut oil

Salt and pepper, to taste

Instructions:

Heat coconut oil in a pot over moderate heat.

Add onion and garlic, sauté until translucent.

Add spinach and cook until wilted.

Pour in vegetable broth and coconut milk.

Bring to a simmer.

Using an immersion blender, mix the soup until it is smooth.

Season with salt and pepper, then serve hot.

Beef and Broccoli Stir-Fry

Ingredients:

1 lb. (450g) beef slices (choose a lean cut)

2 cups broccoli florets

1 tablespoon coconut oil

2 garlic cloves, minced

1/4 cup tamari or coconut aminos

1 teaspoon sesame oil

Salt and pepper, to taste

Instructions:

Heat the coconut oil in a pan over medium-high heat.

Add garlic and beef, cooking until the beef is nearly cooked through.

Add broccoli and tamari (or coconut aminos).

Stir well and cover, letting it steam for about 3-5 minutes.

Drizzle with sesame oil and season with salt and pepper to taste.

Serve hot.

Lemon Garlic Baked Cod

Ingredients:

2 cod fillets

2 tablespoons olive oil

Juice of 1 lemon

2 garlic cloves, minced

1 teaspoon dried thyme

Salt and pepper, to taste

Instructions:

Preheat the oven to 400°F (200°C).

Place cod fillets in a baking dish.

In a small bowl, mix olive oil, lemon juice, garlic, thyme, salt, and pepper.

Pour the mixture over the cod fillets.

Bake for 12-15 minutes or until the cod is flaky and cooked through.

Serve hot.

Eggplant Lasagna

Ingredients:

2 large eggplants, sliced lengthwise

1 cup sugar-free tomato sauce

1 lb. (450g) ground turkey, cooked

1 cup ricotta cheese (or a dairy-free alternative)

1/2 cup grated Parmesan (optional)

1 tablespoon olive oil

Salt and pepper, to taste

Instructions:

Preheat the oven to 375°F (190°C).

Brush eggplant slices with olive oil and season with salt
and pepper.

Grill or roast until tender.

In a baking dish, layer eggplant slices, tomato sauce,
cooked ground turkey, and dollops of ricotta cheese.

Repeat layers.

Top with grated Parmesan, if using.

Bake for 25-30 minutes or until bubbly.

Serve hot.

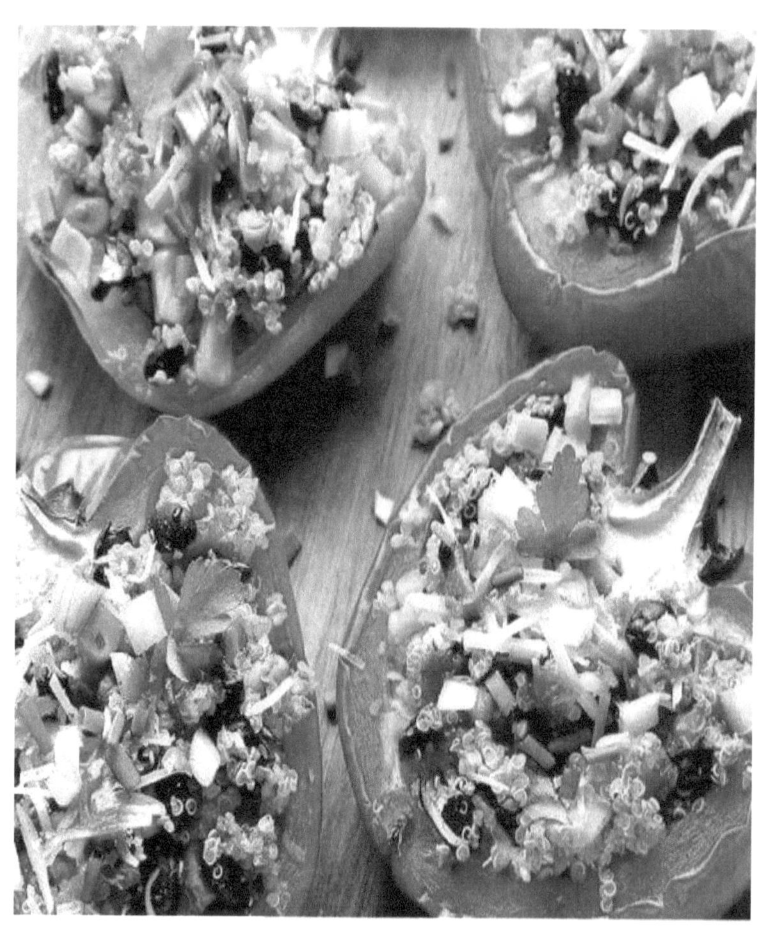

Stuffed Bell Peppers

Ingredients:

4 bell peppers, tops removed and seeded

1 lb. (450g) ground chicken, cooked

1 cup spinach, chopped

1/2 cup diced mushrooms

cup diced onion

1 cup cauliflower rice

1 teaspoon garlic powder

1 teaspoon paprika

Salt and pepper, to taste

1/2 cup sugar-free tomato sauce

Instructions:

Preheat your oven to 375°F (190°C).

In a skillet, cook the ground chicken over medium heat
until browned.

Set aside.

In the same skillet, add a bit more oil if needed, and sauté
the onion, mushrooms, and spinach until soft.

Mix the cooked chicken back into the skillet with the vegetables.

Add the cauliflower rice, garlic powder, paprika, salt, and pepper.

Stir well to combine.

Spoon the mixture into each bell pepper cavity until full.

Place the stuffed peppers in a baking dish.

Pour the tomato sauce over the tops of the stuffed peppers.

Cover with foil and bake for about 30-35 minutes, or until the peppers are tender.

Remove the foil and bake for an additional 5-10 minutes to slightly brown the tops.

Serve hot.

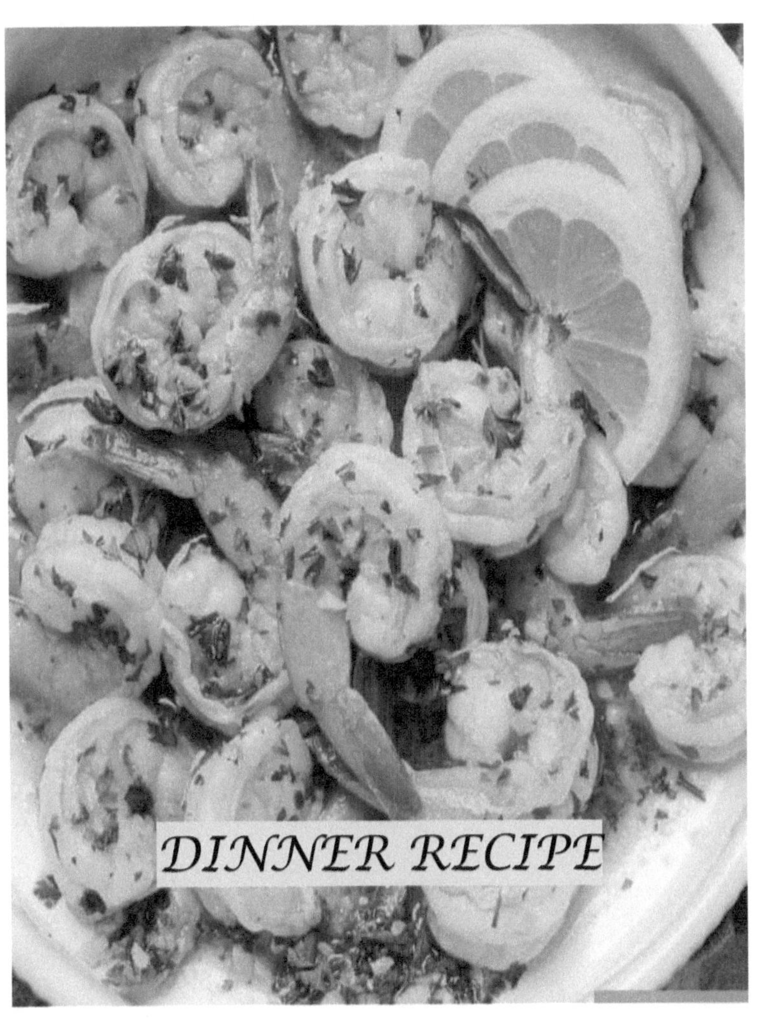
DINNER RECIPE

DINNER RECIPE
Herb-Crusted Salmon

Ingredients:

2 salmon fillets

2 tablespoons olive oil

1 tablespoon fresh dill, chopped

1 tablespoon fresh parsley, chopped

1 garlic clove, minced

Salt and pepper, to taste

Instructions:

Preheat your oven to 400°F (200°C).

Mix olive oil, dill, parsley, garlic, salt, and pepper in a bowl.

Place salmon fillets on a baking sheet lined with parchment paper.

Brush the herb mixture over the salmon fillets.

Bake for 12-15 minutes or until salmon is cooked through.

Lemon Garlic Shrimp

Ingredients:

1 lb. (450g) shrimp, peeled and deveined

3 tablespoons olive oil

Juice of 1 lemon

3 garlic cloves, minced

1 teaspoon paprika

Salt and pepper, to taste

2 tablespoons fresh parsley, chopped

Instructions:

In a large bowl, mix olive oil, lemon juice, garlic, paprika, salt, and pepper.

Add shrimp and marinate for 15-30 minutes.

Heat a skillet over medium-high heat.

Add the shrimp and fry for 2-3 minutes each side.

Garnish with fresh parsley before serving.

Coconut Curry Chicken

Ingredients:

2 chicken breasts, cubed

1 can coconut milk

1 tablespoon coconut oil

1 tablespoon curry powder

1/2 teaspoon turmeric

1 red bell pepper, sliced

1 onion, diced

Salt and pepper, to taste

Instructions:

Heat coconut oil in a large skillet over moderate heat.

Add chicken cubes and cook until browned.

Remove and set aside.

In the same skillet, add onion and bell pepper, cooking until soft.

Return the chicken to the skillet.

Add coconut milk, curry powder, and turmeric.

Simmer for 20 minutes. Season with salt and pepper.

Serve hot.

Zucchini Noodles with Pesto

Ingredients:

4 zucchinis, spiralized

1 cup fresh basil leaves

1/4 cup olive oil

1/4 cup pine nuts

2 garlic cloves

Salt and pepper, to taste

Instructions:

For the pesto, blend basil, olive oil, pine nuts, garlic, salt, and pepper until smooth.

In a pan, lightly sauté zucchini noodles for 2-3 minutes.

Remove from heat and mix in the pesto sauce.

Serve immediately.

Baked Lemon Pepper Chicken

Ingredients:

4 chicken thighs

2 tablespoons olive oil

1 lemon, juiced and zested

1 teaspoon black pepper

Salt, to taste

Instructions:

Preheat your oven to 375°F (190°C).

In a bowl, combine olive oil, lemon juice and zest, pepper, and salt.

Place chicken thighs in a baking dish and coat with the lemon pepper mixture.

Bake for 35-40 minutes or until chicken is fully cooked.

Serve hot.

Stuffed Acorn Squash

Ingredients:

2 acorn squashes, halved and seeds removed

1 lb. (450g) ground turkey

1 tablespoon olive oil

1/2 cup onions, diced

1/2 cup bell peppers, diced

1 teaspoon garlic powder

1 teaspoon dried thyme

Salt and pepper, to taste

Instructions:

Preheat your oven to 400°F (200°C).

Place acorn squash halves face-up on a baking sheet and bake for 25 minutes.

Meanwhile, heat olive oil in a skillet.

Add ground turkey, onions, bell peppers, garlic powder, thyme, salt, and pepper.

Cook until the turkey is browned.

Stuff the turkey mixture into the roasted acorn squash halves and bake for an additional 20 minutes.

Serve warm.

Garlic Butter Mushrooms

Ingredients:

2 cups mushrooms, cleaned

2 tablespoons olive oil

3 garlic cloves, minced

2 tablespoons fresh parsley, chopped

Salt and pepper, to taste

Instructions:

Heat olive oil in a skillet over medium heat.

Add mushrooms and cook for 5 minutes until they start to brown.

Add garlic, salt, and pepper, and cook for another 2 minutes.

Garnish with parsley before serving.

Roasted Brussels Sprouts

Ingredients:

3 cups Brussels sprouts, halved

2 tablespoons olive oil

1 teaspoon garlic powder

Salt and pepper, to taste

Instructions:

Preheat your oven to 400°F (200°C).

Toss the Brussels sprouts with olive oil, garlic powder, salt, and pepper.

Spread on a baking sheet and roast for 25-30 minutes, until crispy.

Serve hot.

Cauliflower Steak

Ingredients:

2 large cauliflower heads

3 tablespoons olive oil

1 teaspoon garlic powder

1 teaspoon smoked paprika

Salt and pepper, to taste

Instructions:

Preheat your oven to 400°F (200°C).

Slice cauliflower heads into 1-inch-thick steaks.

Brush both sides with olive oil and season with garlic powder, smoked paprika, salt, and pepper.

Bake for 25 minutes, flipping halfway through, until tender and golden.

Serve hot.

Eggplant Parmesan (No Breading)

Ingredients:

2 eggplants, sliced into 1/2-inch rounds

2 cups sugar-free marinara sauce

1 cup shredded mozzarella (dairy-free if necessary)

1/4 cup fresh basil leaves

Salt and pepper, to taste

2 tablespoons olive oil

Instructions:

Preheat your oven to 375°F (190°C).

Salt the eggplant slices and let them sit for 20 minutes to draw out moisture.

Rinse and pat dry.

Arrange eggplant slices on a baking sheet, brush with olive oil, and season with pepper.

Bake for 20 minutes, turning once, until gently browned.

In a baking dish, layer marinara sauce, baked eggplant slices, and mozzarella.

Repeat layers.

Bake for another 20 minutes, until the cheese is bubbling and brown.

Garnish with fresh basil before serving.

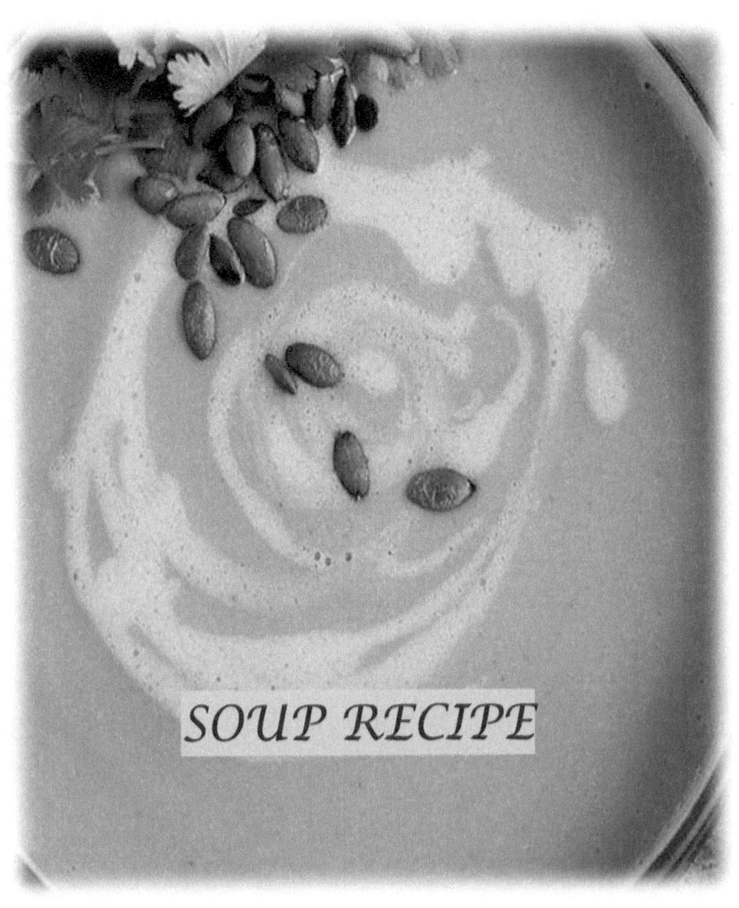

SOUP RECIPE

SOUP RECIPE

Creamy Coconut Ginger Soup

Ingredients:

1 tablespoon coconut oil

1 onion, diced

2 cloves garlic, minced

1 tablespoon ginger, grated

1 carrot, diced

1 stalk celery, diced

1 can coconut milk

4 cups vegetable broth

Salt and pepper, to taste

Fresh cilantro, for garnish

Instructions:

In a large saucepan, melt coconut oil over medium heat.
Sauté the onion, garlic, and ginger until the onion becomes transparent.
Add carrot and celery, and cook for 5 minutes.
Pour in coconut milk and vegetable broth.
Season with salt and pepper.
Bring to a boil, then simmer for 20 minutes.
Blend until smooth using an immersion blender.
Serve garnished with fresh cilantro.

Healing Bone Broth Soup

Ingredients:

2 tablespoons olive oil

1 onion, chopped

2 carrots, chopped

2 stalks celery, chopped

4 cups bone broth

1 teaspoon turmeric

Salt and pepper, to taste

Fresh parsley, for garnish

Instructions:

In a large pot, heat olive oil over moderate heat.

Add onion, carrots, and celery.

Cook until vegetables are soft.

Add bone broth and turmeric.

Season with salt and pepper.

Bring to a boil, then let it simmer for 30 minutes.

Serve garnished with fresh parsley.

Detoxifying Lemon Vegetable Soup

Ingredients:

2 tablespoons olive oil

1 onion, diced

2 cloves garlic, minced

2 zucchinis, diced

2 cups spinach

4 cups vegetable broth

Juice of 1 lemon

Salt and pepper, to taste

Instructions:

In a large saucepan, heat the olive oil over medium heat.

Sauté the onion and garlic until they are transparent.

Add zucchinis and cook for 5 minutes.

Add spinach and vegetable broth.

Bring to a boil, then reduce heat and let to simmer for 10 minutes.

Add lemon juice and season with salt and pepper.

Serve hot.

Spicy Tomato and Basil Soup

Ingredients:

1 tablespoon olive oil

1 onion, diced

2 cloves garlic, minced

1 can (14 oz) diced tomatoes

2 cups vegetable broth

1 teaspoon red pepper flakes (adjust to taste)

1 cup fresh basil, chopped

Salt and pepper, to taste

Instructions:

In a medium-size saucepan, heat the olive oil.

Add the onion and garlic and cook until tender.

Combine the chopped tomatoes (with juice), vegetable broth, and red pepper flakes.

Bring to a boil, then decrease the heat and simmer for 20 minutes.

Add basil and purée the soup with an immersion blender until smooth.

Season with salt and pepper. Serve hot.

Broccoli Almond Soup

Ingredients:

2 tablespoons olive oil

1 onion, diced

1 stalk celery, chopped

4 cups broccoli florets

4 cups vegetable broth

1/2 cup raw almonds

Salt and pepper, to taste

Instructions:

In a large pot, heat olive oil over moderate heat.

Sauté onion and celery until softened.

Add broccoli and vegetable broth.

Bring to a boil, then reduce heat and let to simmer for 15 minutes.

Add almonds, and blend the soup until smooth using an immersion blender.

Season with salt and pepper.

Serve hot.

Cucumber Dill Soup

Ingredients:

2 large cucumbers, peeled and chopped

2 tablespoons olive oil

1 onion, diced

4 cups vegetable broth

1/4 cup fresh dill, chopped

Salt and pepper, to taste

1/2 cup coconut cream

Instructions:

In a pot, heat olive oil over moderate heat.

Add onion and cook until translucent.

Add cucumbers and cook for 5 minutes.

Pour in vegetable broth and bring to a simmer for 10 minutes.

Stir in dill and coconut cream.

Blend until smooth.

Season with salt and pepper.

Chill before serving.

Carrot Ginger Soup

Ingredients:

2 tablespoons coconut oil

1 onion, diced

2 cloves garlic, minced

2 tablespoons fresh ginger, minced

6 carrots, peeled and chopped

4 cups vegetable broth

Salt and pepper, to taste

Instructions:

In a large pot, heat coconut oil over moderate heat.

Add onion, garlic, and ginger, cooking until onion is soft.

Add carrots and vegetable broth.

Bring to a boil, then reduce heat and simmer for about 20

minutes, or until carrots are soft.

Use an immersion blender to smooth up the soup.

Season with salt and pepper to taste.

Serve hot.

Creamy Avocado Soup

Ingredients:

2 ripe avocados, pitted and scooped

1 cucumber, peeled and chopped

1 tablespoon lime juice

2 cups vegetable broth, chilled

1 garlic clove, minced

Salt and pepper, to taste

Fresh cilantro, for garnish

Instructions:

Blend avocados, cucumber, lime juice, vegetable broth, and garlic until smooth.

Season with salt and pepper to taste.

Chill for at least one hour before serving.

Garnish with fresh cilantro.

Roasted Red Pepper and Tomato Soup

Ingredients:

2 tablespoons olive oil

1 onion, diced

2 cloves garlic, minced

1 jar (12 oz) roasted red peppers, drained and chopped

1 can (14 oz) diced tomatoes

4 cups vegetable broth

Salt and pepper, to taste

Fresh basil, for garnish

Instructions:

In a medium-size saucepan, heat the olive oil.

Add the onion and garlic and heat until softened.

Combine the roasted red peppers and chopped tomatoes.

Cook for five minutes.

Bring the vegetable broth to a boil for 20 minutes.

Blend the soup until smooth. Season with salt and pepper.

Serve garnished with fresh basil.

Spinach and Asparagus Soup

Ingredients:

2 tablespoons olive oil

1 onion, diced

2 cloves garlic, minced

1 bunch asparagus, trimmed and chopped

4 cups spinach leaves

4 cups vegetable broth

Salt and pepper, to taste

Lemon zest, for garnish

Instructions:

In a large saucepan, heat the olive oil over medium heat.

Add the onion and garlic and sauté until transparent.

Add asparagus and cook for 5 minutes.

Add spinach and vegetable broth.

Bring to a boil, then simmer for 10 minutes or until asparagus is tender.

Use an immersion blender to carefully blend the soup until smooth.

Season with salt and pepper to taste.

Serve hot, garnished with lemon zest for a refreshing twist.

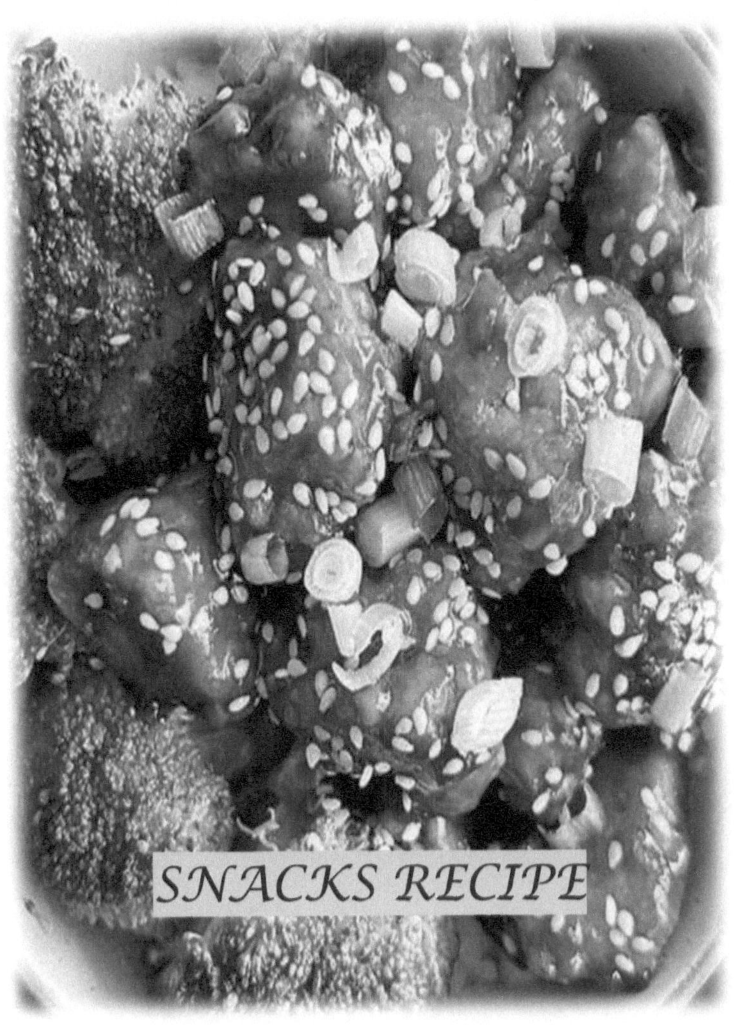
SNACKS RECIPE

SNACKS RECIPE
Avocado Lime Snack

Ingredients:

1 ripe avocado

Juice of 1 lime

A pinch of sea salt

A sprinkle of chili flakes (optional)

Instructions:

Halve the avocado and remove the pit.

Drizzle lime juice over each half.

Sprinkle with sea salt and chili flakes.

Enjoy with a spoon directly from the skin.

Coconut Yogurt with Cinnamon

Ingredients:

1 cup unsweetened coconut yogurt

1/2 teaspoon cinnamon

Instructions:

Mix the coconut yogurt with cinnamon.

Serve chilled as a creamy, dairy-free snack.

Cucumber and Herb Salad

Ingredients:

2 large cucumbers, thinly sliced

2 tablespoons olive oil

1 tablespoon apple cider vinegar

Fresh dill, chopped

Salt and pepper to taste

Instructions:

Toss cucumber slices with olive oil, apple cider vinegar, and fresh dill.

Season with salt and pepper.

Chill for 10 minutes before serving.

Almond Butter Celery Sticks

Ingredients:

Celery sticks

Almond butter

Instructions:

Spread almond butter generously inside the groove of each celery stick.

Enjoy as a crunchy and creamy snack.

Roasted Pumpkin Seeds

Ingredients:

1 cup raw pumpkin seeds
1 tablespoon olive oil
A pinch of sea salt

Instructions:

Preheat oven to 300°F (150°C).

Toss pumpkin seeds with olive oil and sea salt.

Spread on a baking sheet and roast for about 45 minutes, stirring occasionally until golden and crunchy.

Zucchini Chips

Ingredients:

2 zucchinis

Olive oil spray

Sea salt

Instructions:

Preheat oven to 225°F (105°C).

Slice zucchinis thinly and lay out on a baking sheet lined with parchment paper.

Spray lightly with olive oil and sprinkle with sea salt.

Bake for 2 hours or until crisp, turning halfway through.

Garlic Stuffed Olives

Ingredients:

1 cup green olives, pitted

2 cloves garlic, thinly sliced

1 tablespoon olive oil

1 teaspoon dried oregano

Instructions:

Stuff each olive with a slice of garlic.

Toss olives with olive oil and oregano.

Marinate for at least 30 minutes before serving.

Coconut Almond Energy Balls

Ingredients:

1 cup almond flour

1/2 cup shredded unsweetened coconut

1/4 cup coconut oil, melted

1 tablespoon xylitol or erythritol

Instructions:

Mix all ingredients in a bowl until well combined.

Roll into small balls and refrigerate until firm.

Lemon Pepper Kale Chips

Ingredients:

1 bunch kale, washed and dried

1 tablespoon olive oil

1 teaspoon lemon zest

Black pepper to taste

Instructions:

Preheat oven to 300°F (150°C).

Tear kale into bite-sized pieces and toss with olive oil,

lemon zest, and black pepper.

Bake for 15 minutes or until crisp.

Herb-Infused Mixed Nuts

Ingredients:

2 cups mixed nuts (almonds, walnuts, pecans)

1 tablespoon olive oil

1 teaspoon rosemary, finely chopped

1 teaspoon thyme, finely chopped

Sea salt to taste

Instructions:

Preheat oven to 350°F (175°C).

Toss nuts with olive oil, rosemary, thyme, and sea salt.

Spread on a baking sheet and roast for 10-15 minutes,

stirring occasionally.

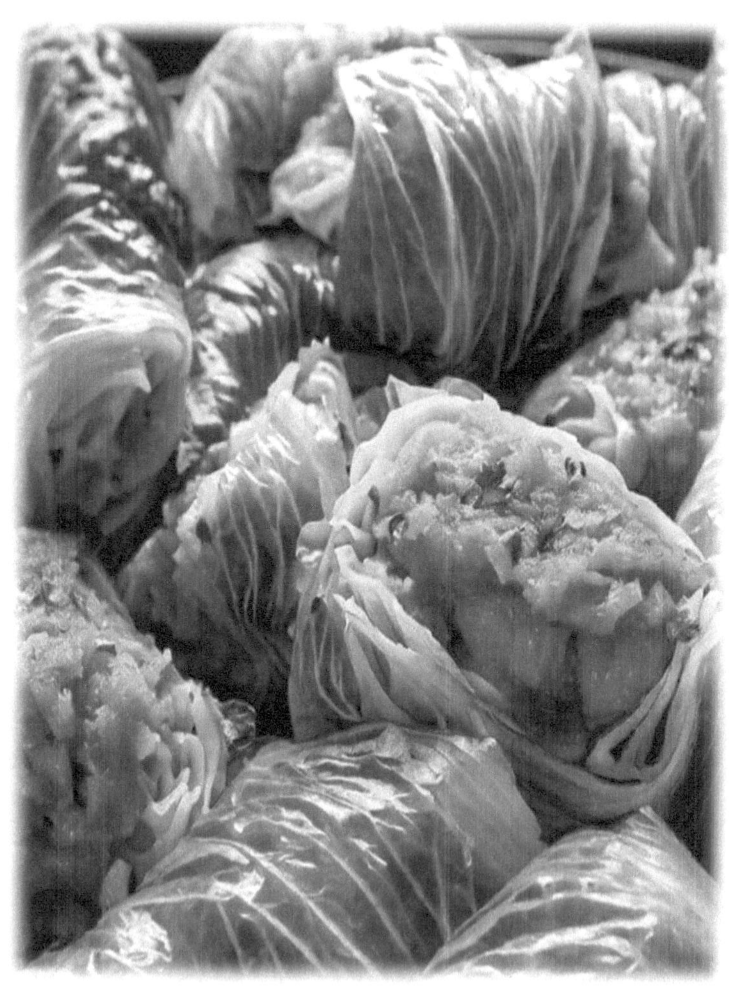

CONCLUSION

This collection of recipes is more than just a compilation of meals; it represents a holistic approach to wellness, emphasizing the power of whole foods, balanced nutrition, and mindful eating.

Our exploration began with breakfast, the foundation of daily nutrition, where we introduced meals that energize the body without feeding Candida. Lunch recipes followed, offering sustaining and flavorful dishes that carry you through the day. Dinner options were crafted to not only satisfy but also to support a healing environment for your body overnight. Soups brought comfort and healing nutrients in a bowl, while snacks provided safe and tasty options for those moments in between meals.

Each recipe was carefully developed with the dual goals of combating Candida overgrowth and promoting overall health. By prioritizing ingredients that are low in sugars and rich in nutrients, we aimed to equip you with a toolkit not just for dietary management, but for a lifestyle transformation.

Candida overgrowth can be a challenging condition, affecting not just physical health but also emotional well-being. Through these pages, we've sought to offer not just a diet, but a lifeline: a means to reclaim control over your health, one meal at a time.

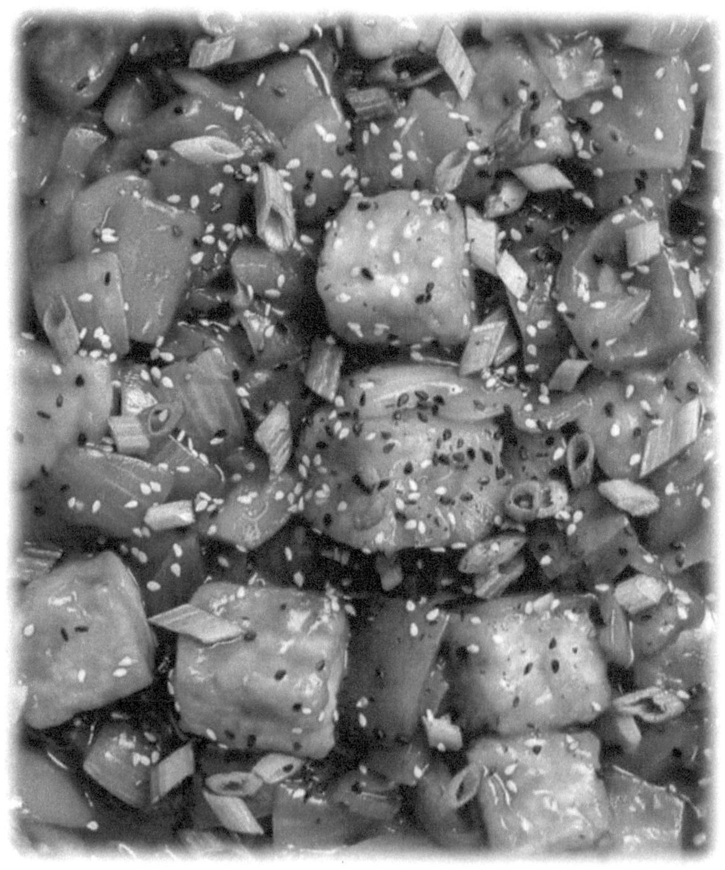

www.ingramcontent.com/pod-product-compliance
Lightning Source LLC
Chambersburg PA
CBHW031329250726
48656CB00005B/2046